Advance Praise

"This book is fantastic. I could not put it down! And it is exactly what has worked for me, while working with Abby. I highly recommend it."

—**Sandi Hintz**, long-time client of the Ortho Healing Center

"*Reverse Button* is well-written, and the recollection of so many client experiences is amazing. By reading excerpts to my husband, he now understands my reasoning for spending time and money with Ortho Healing Center rather than so many medical facilities. I fully agree that specialization has left a gap in the rehabilitation of the human body. So much is lost between facilities and doctors. Even with the software used to share information of patient history, little time is spent by the specialists to read that which is available. We must advocate for ourselves and demand alternative tests and treatments in order to alleviate our pain. Yes, there are times in which surgery is necessary; however, *Reverse Button* provides a much more humanistic approach to healing."

> —**Ellie deBrauwere**, Attendee of the first Reverse Button 3-day Intensive Retreat

"Abby's knowledge pool is both deep and wide. In *Reverse Button*, she has distilled her reservoir of experience into a cup full of sweet water that anyone can drink from and find comfort for both body and soul. I understand that my body knows far more than my mind can comprehend about myself and so many other things. Yet I have not trusted that I could hear its messages accurately. Through these pages, I have come to trust that my body will let me know what it needs and that I will choose to listen and respond well, whether the message is about food, or activities, or who it wants to be around."

> —**Vienna**, author of *Your Hands On Manual for Neck and Back Relief*

"Abby doesn't operate on protocol. She is very present with every contact experience with the client and what is 'up' for them in that moment, on that day. Her knowledge of and access to the therapeutic techniques are very skilled. I found more tools for self-care and awareness. I have a deeper appreciation for my body now! I loved the sharing of so many stories. I got way more than I anticipated. A lot of information! I feel really empowered and present!"

—**Dena Baron**, attendee of the first
Reverse Button Retreat

REVERSE BUTTON

REVERSE BUTTON™

Learn What the
Doctors **AREN'T**
Telling You,
**AVOID BACK
SURGERY,**
and Get Your
FULL Life Back

Abby Beauchamp

NEW YORK

LONDON • NASHVILLE • MELBOURNE • VANCOUVER

Reverse Button™

Learn What the Doctors Aren't Telling You, Avoid Back Surgery, and Get Your Full Life Back

Published in New York, New York, by Morgan James Publishing in partnership with Difference Press. Morgan James is a trademark of Morgan James, LLC. www.MorganJamesPublishing.com

ISBN 9781642797428 paperback
ISBN 9781642797435 eBook
ISBN 9781642797442 audiobook
Library of Congress Control Number: 2019948184

Cover Design by:
Rachel Lopez
www.r2cdesign.com

Interior Design by:
Christopher Kirk
www.GFSstudio.com

Ortho-Bionomy® is a registered trademark of the Society of Ortho-Bionomy International, Inc. and is used with permission.

Any representative of the Ortho Healing Center or Ortho Healing, LLC is legally not allowed to prescribe or diagnose a health condition. They are, however, allowed to share stories of products or services that have supported their own or others return to comfort and function. It is up to you to do your due diligence and speak with your doctor.

Any statements made by either Seacret Direct (the "Company") or independent "Agents" of the Company, regarding Seacret products, have not been evaluated by the US Food and Drug Administration ("FDA"). Seacret Products are not intended to diagnose, treat, cure, or prevent any disease.

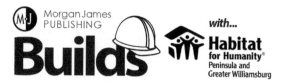

Morgan James is a proud partner of Habitat for Humanity Peninsula and Greater Williamsburg. Partners in building since 2006.

Get involved today! Visit
MorganJamesPublishing.com/giving-back

To Christie Gregg, my ideal reader character,
whom I created out of a collection of my friends
and clients that I wrote this book for to help
them get back to fully living their life again!

Table of Contents

For the Person Looking to Fully Regain their Whole Life Back

When deciding to write this book, I sat with my client list. While people come to see me for all sorts of reasons, the one that rose to the top was to avoid a surgery; particularly back surgery. Generally, it was a mature, successful woman who was doing all she could to manage all that she had going in her life with her career, family, friends, charity, etc. The pain was robbing her from being involved with these aspects of her life she cared the most about. Working through trying to get rid of the pain was becoming very expensive and time consuming; however, what is the alternative? She gives up and just accepts that she will not get to enjoy her life fully. This is just part of aging. She takes months off and goes into a surgery that may or may not actually correct the problem and brings many other risk factors into consideration, including the medications that would be prescribed. It all can be so overwhelming and depressing, and especially hard to work through when the pain is so great in your back you feel you are either going to snap like a rubber band or be collapsed into a permanent fetal position.

A few months ago, I had a client who came to me with the diagnosis of fibromyalgia, chronic fatigue, and a lifetime of pain. It had become her norm. She had done her absolute best to work with it as part of her life; like a relative that needs to be there but you don't really like much. She had raised her family, had success in business, and wanted to enjoy her grandkids, but the pain was always present. The one thing she hadn't tried up to this point was a treatment at the Ortho Healing Center with me. She made the appointment, not fully knowing what to expect and without too much faith that things would change. She just needed to take the edge off, she said. After about forty-five minutes of working together, she slowly got up off the table and politely thanked me. I explained that I'd love to see her again in about seven to ten days to see what the body did with the information in the first three days and whether it was able to hold or not. Again, she nodded politely, but I knew she wasn't really confident much would change. However, she did make the second appointment. When she walked in about a week later, she had the biggest smile on her face! "I am eighty percent better!" she said. I stopped her and really had us both take those words in.

This is a woman who had been in pain for decades. Eighty percent better!

She said her family commented that she was interacting differently with them, and she wasn't quite sure how she felt about that. I asked her to explain what she meant, and she said the family said she was calmer. As she told me more, we figured out that this new feeling of life without the pain would give her the ability to relate to the world in a way she had long forgotten was a possibility … that her body found a comfort and function that she had forgotten was still in there! By working together, we found her Reverse Button™!

Years ago on Facebook, I saw a picture with a stick figure talking to another stick figure that had an explosion of thought bubbles and color coming from its head. The first one was asking, "What is that?" The second one said,

"Oh, it's just my mind." When we learn about something new, especially something that challenges everything we have been taught, we can truly have our minds blown! It is my hope that this is exactly what happens for you when you read this book! I see it in my practice regularly and feel humbled and honored to be a witness of what the body can do to get back to comfort and function. It excites me to the edge of my existence when a client, like the story above, gets to experience the power behind their amazing body. A moment when everything changes and she has hope and belief again in the power of her body; a true mind blow! Years ago, I read a book together with friends over a retreat weekend called Queen of Your Own Life by Cindy Ratzlaff and Kathy Kinney. The biggest takeaway from this was at the end of the book and the end of the weekend, we had all evaluated what beliefs were serving us and that we would take forward, and what beliefs were not and that we left at that lake that weekend. Our minds were blown. We were forever changed and crowned Queens of Our Own Lives!

Studies have shown the three most important factors for longevity are: community, science-based nutrition, and walking! Community to me is developed in many ways, including finding a person or team to support your body in working in its best function, so you can focus on eating well and getting the exercise you need. I know that when you are being crushed by back pain, the last thing you want to focus on is your food and exercise. My goodness, you are just trying to survive day to day. And I'm here to tell you: you deserve a medal for all you have done to get here! I am confident this is not the first step you have taken to get rid of your back pain. I am deeply grateful you have found this book and that I have the opportunity now to share new information with you; to be a part of your team and community to support you in living your best life of comfort and function! It's an honor to be a contribution that helps you be able to enjoy your kids, grandkids, partner, work, hobbies, charity, and all your other communities that are needed to have a full life!

Right now, I am watching a friend of mine have this exact story unfold in her life. While I'm already a part of her community, her tribe, as her friend she has not decided yet to fully walk through the doors of what I have to offer; she is collapsing day by day from the pain in her back. Disease is starting to take over and I am deeply concerned for her. So why hasn't she fully committed to allowing me to be a part of her health team? It's because she is not ready to believe yet that it can get better. She wants to hold the belief that it has to be something external that is happening to her that can be fixed by an MRI or a magic pill. She is terrified of the thought of surgery. Yet, there is also comfort in receiving the news that someone recognizes just how bad this feels and of course you need surgery because you are suffering. And just maybe if I'm down for months, the community I take care of will be forced to step up and take care of me for once. I recognize this in her and while I worry about her daily; it is a journey we each need to take. I have deep compassion for her journey or her timing and absolutely don't take it personally. If you are at this same point; know it is ok; save this book for later or pass it on to someone who is ready to have new information downloaded and who is ready to decide that she can live her whole life again without pain and without surgery! If we work together, I will acknowledge your pain, have deep compassion and caring for you, and I will hold the possibility that you can regain your full life back! Your pain is real! Your timing of when you are ready to let it go and believe there is a Reverse Button in your body waiting to be pushed back to a time of better comfort and function is your timing! If that timing is now, I am thrilled to welcome you to the Ortho Healing Center, Ortho-Bionomy®, Intuitive Healing Facilitation, molecular hydrogen, vagus nerve, and other weird words I will go into depth in this book together with you. I welcome you to my tribe and have deep gratitude that you have chosen to explore this option for you! Let's find your Reverse Button today!

As a gift for you, I have put together bonus content of one-page quick reference sheets and short videos I will share with you as a thank you for going on this journey with me. Just email: ReverseButtonBook@gmail.com with the subject: "Bonus Content." Now let's get started.

CHAPTER

2

My Story

So, the last thing I thought I would ever do in the world is touch people for a living! Some of my previous jobs were working at the Department of Revenue and owning a Montessori School. These are not touching-people jobs; it's pretty much against the rules. But to understand why I understand your journey and how I've come to help so many find their way back to their comfort and function, I need to tell you a few things about myself first.

Most of my childhood, I was labeled "the klutz" and "overly sensitive." I never seemed to know where my body was at, and I ran into things constantly. My dad even asked me one time if it was possible for me to make it through a doorway without being hurt. I seriously questioned it.

Growing up poor in Southern Oregon without insurance, my mother's superpower was creativity – including in our healthcare. To this day, I still don't understand why if I got strep throat, I went to the dentist for antibiotics instead of a doctor. We saw an osteopath as our primary care provider because he was cheaper than an MD. My aunt studied to be a shaman and opened my eyes at a young age to other ways to help a body than the healthcare system all my friends used.

When I was seventeen, I was going to lunch with a friend, sitting sideways in the passenger seat and chatting away when another car load of teenagers decided to flip a U-turn too fast and didn't see us. They plowed into the passenger side of the car. The seat belt came down hard and fast. My pelvis was flattened. The doctors would later tell me that most likely I would never be able to carry a baby to term. I would walk and my leg would slip out of joint; I would have to find a step and push it back in, otherwise I would drag it. I saw Chiropractors, Massage Therapists, BioFeedback Specialists, Osteopaths, and more. For ten years, I drug a leg, and bodywork became a regular budget line for me to maintain any level of function.

Also, at the ripe old age of seventeen, my mother and I got in the biggest fight of that time and I ran away from home. OK, I was gone less than twenty-four hours, but it was a big deal in my mind. It was also the catalyst that started me down the path of seeing a counselor and starting to really learn more about myself and the human condition. The biggest recurring theme in counseling was that I needed better boundaries and that I was a very sensitive person. Both comments felt very shaming, and just like with all the bodywork I received, I maintained but didn't make it back over the hump to what I now know to be comfort and function.

Three more car accidents and two children later (lucky the doctors were wrong about my ability to carry a baby), I was still having regular mental support and bodywork from my collection of my care team. In the care team I found an incredible massage therapist named Sandra that really started me with my first understanding that sometimes you need to work somewhere else in the body then what was obvious. And sometimes the problem has to do with your management of stress in your life. She had noticed that when I was stressed my shoulders would shrug up and that the muscle connected from my shoulder blade to my hip would pull my hip out of socket. Instead of working on my lower body like everyone else, she wanted to just focus on the upper half of my body for a while and see what would happen. I went in every week for almost a year and my pelvis stabilized. It was *amazing!* My body was able to self-correct when I set the environment up for it to do so.

Just as I was able to get my pelvis to stabilize a bit and stop dragging a leg, and all was at a calm place in my life … my body had a complete meltdown. Some call this part of a healing journey. I felt like someone flipped a switch inside, and in a matter of one month, I was having seizures, drop-outs (sort of opposite of a seizure where everything slows down – like your heart and lungs), hot flashes, night sweats, and migraines. I wasn't able to drive for nearly a year and a half while I went from doctor to doctor. No one could figure out anything for me. I learned to become my own advocate.

During my first pregnancy, I had completely gone in the opposite direction from my childhood and jumped fully into the medical system. I did most everything my doctors recommended for me and my child. Almost five years later, I had my second child and had done a lot of reading. I was eating whole, organic, seasonal foods. Using natural remedies for my healthcare, I had moved my primary care provider to a naturopath and chosen an alternative immunization plan for my daughter. I swung the opposite direction on the healthcare spectrum. Through all of this, I learned there is a need for both natural care and medical intervention, but in the end, I am my best advocate. I am the one who lives in this body and knows it better than anyone else. I am the one that needs to offer it an environment to do its very best, so it can find its best comfort and function. I need to trust and believe that my body is intelligent and wants to go forward in comfort and function too. We are a team and are in this together! Things like migraines as frequent as every two weeks for eight years is ridiculous! My body was *screaming* at me that I needed to listen to it, and instead, I would self-medicate or decide I could be tough and get past it. Looking back, I have had to apologize to my body many times. Pain is there for communication. Waiting till you are diagnosed with PTSD, adrenal fatigue, cortisol flooding, and more means you are buying into the belief that "pain is gain." If you just keep working faster, then you can be tough enough to get past this. My friend, this is not true. We need to honor this beautiful system that is here wanting to work with you. It's not against you. This is one of my biggest lessons to date and if you only take one thing away from this book, I hope this is it! Your body wants to work in comfort and function. It wants to work with you!

Flash forward several years, and the Montessori School I had was closed due to the economy drop in 2008. I was suddenly in between careers. I was focused on being a mom who volunteered at the kids' school for everything, learned how to garden and preserve food, and helped out with the books of my family business. Then my sister-in-law came home for a visit from Colorado. She declared that she was giving up her Commercial Contractor business and was going to become an Ortho-Bionomist, and suggested that I should, too. I think I actually laughed out loud. Me, touch someone for a living? That would just be silly. If my own husband had a sore neck, I would send him to the massage therapist, as a good wife should!

She was nice and left me alone for a short time. Then she called from New Mexico. She had just found out that there was a weekend class for horse and rider that had no prerequisites and that I should come down and take it with her. When she had been home last, I had told her about a horse that had come into my daughter's barn that I had fallen in love with. I had fallen so in love, in fact, that I convinced my husband that I needed to pre-pay thousands of dollars for energetic groundwork lessons with this horse so my friend could actually buy it and give me regular access to it. This horse was sold to my friend as one "who needed a firm hand" because she had kicked a child. They said she probably shouldn't be around any women or children. Both the previous owners and my friend spent a lot of time with Splash to try to help her find her happy place again, but this horse and I needed each other to do that. I wasn't a horse person before, but this horse had a hold of my heart and I would do anything for her. With that said, I took a look at the points on my credit card and had within five points to get my hotel and airfare. So, I got on a plane to New Mexico to help a horse.

When I arrived in New Mexico, I was *so* far out of my comfort zone. This class was eight hours on people and eight hours working on horses. It was made up of serious horse women who knew their way around. I didn't want to tell them about my lack of horse knowledge, but they figured it out pretty quickly. Everyone was very kind in helping me find my way. I ended up pairing up with a young woman who had been on horses and fallen off horses her entire life. They told us about the spine and had us feel the curvature in each other's spines. I could have put a two by four board up against her back because it was so straight – no curve at all! Then, I was to put her on a massage table and gently lift her leg, just until the hip point softened, put a gentle compression in and wait for about ten seconds and gently put the leg back down. They had us re-check the spine. Hers now looked like the skeleton model in the room.

How was that possible? I had had many bodyworkers in my life and I had never seen a body correct that quickly. This was her first class, too, and she was absolutely blown away. All weekend we would re-check to see if it was holding – and it did! At the end of the first day of class, I told my sister-in-law that it felt like the first time I ever went into a Montessori classroom. I didn't know what they were doing that was so different, I could just feel it was different and I was intrigued. I needed to learn more!

I went back home and all I could remember was how to work on the hoof, so in six weeks, I gave Splash four treatments and she was a transformed horse! She loved life again. She loved it so much that for years the only time she really needed any significant work was when she was enjoying herself too much in the field and slipped or ran into a gate … or sometimes she was having so much fun that another horse would kick and correct her. She inspired me regularly to find the daily joy in life!

The instructor I had at the Ortho-Bionomy class was a woman from Australia. She told stories of her ranch she owned there and how she would take several months of the year and travel across the US to teach. I thought this sounded like the most amazing job ever! I wanted to become an Instructor! Sadly, I found out for that year she was done teaching in the US. If I wanted any more classes from her, I would have to go to Australia. As tempting as that was, I decided to just find out what the next available Ortho class was in the US. It happened to be in Grand Junction, Colorado with a woman named Sheri Covey. My sister-in-law had told Sheri that I had taken energetic groundwork classes for horses and this one Ortho class and so I would be able to keep up with a very energetic advanced class called Chapman's Reflexes. She arranged drinks the night before class for Sheri and me to meet.

I will never forget that moment. Sheri explained to me that in Ortho, she would teach me how to meet energy and then come back away from it. She used her hands to demonstrate the closeness of touch but not merging. A tear ran down my cheek, and I thought, "Is that possible?" So many years of shame that I didn't have good boundaries, so many books read trying to improve my skills, and it that one moment she gave me hope that I felt I could actually find my boundaries!

Sheri shared that she was opening a new school in Denver called the Rocky Mountain Ortho-Bionomy Center, and that I should be part of her first class. The program she had created was ten modules of about a week each, spread out a little over two years. I signed up and she told me she would help me to convert the work to the horses. Over that next two years, I flew to Denver about every six weeks for a module, and then would come home and practice with a herd of seven horses and any friends who would let me. I also spread out and took classes from a dozen of other instructors to get a broader sense of the work. I learned a lot by doing this! While I had a lot of experience with a wide variety of modalities of care, it got really clear to me that every practitioner out there, no matter the work, brought their unique self to flavor their work. They adjusted their lens to offer the world their unique offering to support the common good. I learned to appreciate these differences and to start looking for my own unique gifts.

My kids' school allowed me to set up shop and offer free practice sessions to parents and staff. This was such a gift. Most staff only had fifteen to twenty minutes for me to work with them. So many Ortho practitioners I had worked with were either massage therapists first or influenced by the massage model of focusing on a certain amount of time the body was being touched. This opportunity expanded my understanding of what was possible in even a very short amount of time with a body! I had clients who were seeing a list of care providers, like I used to: chiropractors, massage therapists, physical therapists, etcetera, start saying they loved to pop in for just a few minutes with me and I could be their "one stop shop."

A friend then asked if I would like to come share space with an acupuncturist in her Natural Health Clinic. What a tremendous gift! To work in a thriving, bustling, office with eight different modalities felt so grown up and real! I had to book clients in every sixty minutes, do their intake, and have departure all in that time range. It was fast paced. I was able to experience working very collaboratively with other modalities and practitioners who shared clients. Recognizing each of our gifts that we could share with the clients and that some do need information from more than one direction. I learned and grew so much there and will forever be thankful for that gift of an experience.

While working on finishing up my schooling, I contacted the State of Oregon to find out what I needed to be legal to touch people. I was told either I went to school to get a recognized touch license, like massage and then just blend the two works; or I could work to get the laws changed. Since two things were true: One, I was comfortable with administrative law language thanks to my time in Department of Revenue, and two, I am highly dyslexic and so the thought of the rote memorization of all the muscles and the brutal, on-the-spot massage board test terrified me

… I went with getting the laws changed. It took about a year and a half of monthly meetings in Salem to get the job done. Today Ortho-Bionomists are recognized as their own stand-alone modality, different than anything else in the state and that is safe for Oregonians as long as we hold a practitioner or above license from the Society of Ortho-Bionomy International.

May of 2012, I got to hang my shingle out of my first office in Milwaukie, Oregon. The Ortho Healing Center was born. My sister owned a sign shop at that time and I had her create a logo for me using a favorite photograph of a mandala of leaves and flowers. For the business initials I had a dream of the "O" in a spiral that was represented Splash's front leg when it was being lifted for me to work with. I left the "H" up to her. She did such a great job of turning it into the trees of my property that meant so much to me. The "H" also branched out like the four directions of energetic flow which I later learned. It was perfect. It was red and black because those were the only colors in my wardrobe. The week before I was to open my office, I went to the Portland Mind, Body and Spirit Expo to see if it would be an event to get a booth at in the future. I walked around for about two hours and finally kept coming back to the same booth that was taking pictures of people's auras. They were telling every person different things, so I decided it seemed legit. The man took my money and had me put my hands on his machine. He sat in silence for a moment. He then said, "How are you doing this?"

"Doing what?" I asked.

"How are you in a meditative state?"

I answered, "You mean Ortho-Bionomy?"

He said, "No – what are you doing to maintain your meditative state?"

I said, more confidently, this time, "Ortho-Bionomy. I practice about six to eight hours a day to stay quiet within myself to listen to others."

He proceeded with the reading. He explained that was I surrounded with a lot of blue, which represented that I had enough ability for me to heal myself and others. Then he pointed to the green and said, "You really enjoy helping others and they are very drawn to you for help." He paused dramatically and quietly said, "See the fuchsia?"

It was woven throughout the blue. I said, "Yes."

He looked me directly in the eyes and said, "You can feel everyone in this room, can't you?"

I sheepishly replied, "Yes."

He handed me back most of my money and said, "All I can tell you is to take good care of yourself."

I walked away with my picture, thinking, "Wow, I think I just got gold stars for my aura!" I called my sister and told her to change the logo right away. The new colors of the clinic were to be blue, green, and fuchsia: for healing, intuition, and helping others. My closet diversified its colors too.

With the opening of the clinic, I was very clear that it was an education center before an individual practice. I wanted to empower all to live a life of comfort and function and believed deeply that came through education of all aspects of life from mind, body, spirit, financial, etc. I also felt it meant the clinic was meant to help other Ortho-Bionomy students develop by having a place to do their practice hours. By adding the Student Clinic, it provided a lower cost option for clients who needed it, and funds that could be used to pay directly for students to take more classes, truly a win-win-win scenario. The clinic became to be known as the Ortho Healing Center and Student Clinic for Humans, Dogs, and Horses. My reputation was growing of my individual gifts and many of my clients started to call me the human MRI. One of my favorite moments was when a client opened my office door and blurted out, "I'm pregnant!" She wanted to be able to tell me first, because she knew as soon as I touched her, I would know. I was humbled and laughed out loud! We quickly expanded and moved to a big office with four treatment rooms on Sunnyside Road in Clackamas, Oregon.

The Sunnyside office was growing quickly and from the beginning we were covering our nearly $3,000 in overhead from the start. During this year, my oldest daughter started to struggle with her health and a brain injury was discovered. We learned a lot that year in returning her to her health, and once again I was so grateful to learn that a collaboration was needed for her to return to health. We needed to address her diet, her exercise, and she needed regular cranial bodywork support. At the end of the year, she got her dream to attend a boarding school in France and graduate from a high school in Europe. When I got back from dropping her off at the school in Paris, my husband of sixteen years decided that it was time to let our marriage go. With one child out of the house and my practice flowing, he felt I could make it on my own. Today, I tell this story and know that he was the brave one who said it first. I had been thinking about it for years. I had slept in a separate bedroom for two years. We were partners in the business of the family but that was it. We really ran in two totally different paths of desires in life. We each deserved to find someone who wanted to be on our same path. We committed to not tear each other down and to figure out a way that was as fair as possible for each to start their own separate life.

I bought a large house that my office could move to, I could live in, and that had a rental attached for a second income. This house was extra special because I had a dream about it a year and a half before. This dream was so vivid it scared me, and I talked with so many friends about it. I thought the house was in England because it was a brick Tudor house. It wasn't something I had never been attracted to previously. In the dream, it was so real that it was "my house." I had no sense of where my family was. Just that I lived there with my dog and worked there, too. There was a big house and a little house with a small yard that connected them and it was all surrounded by large hedges.

When I first started to look for houses, I took my dear friend Joni with me. She is significantly older than me, has many rentals and lived alone for many years. I started with condos. I told her I just needed simple after so many years on acreage. She said no, I needed an income property. I told the real estate agent that I could look at those too. The first two places I looked at and started to try to figure out if they made sense, I would hear a voice in my head, "look for the hedges." The voice got louder and more insistent.

The third income property I was taken to was on a corner of two common streets, easy to get to and surrounded by a very old arborvitae hedge. The yard was all nearly parking spaces with an easy pull through drive. I was drawn into the brick Tudor house (I did not associate it with my dream from a year and a half ago during this first look). I walked into a very staged house and met a lovely couple that was retiring and moving into an RV. I loved all the creative touches from the way the walls were painted dark brown and sage green. The staircase with scrolling spiral metalwork blew me away. They proceeded to show me the garden box window in the kitchen. The claw-foot bathtub. The hot tub deck with French doors in the master suite with direct access. Even the furniture was something I would choose. I commented about how perfect it was and they said, "We are happy to sell all the furniture, it would be a gift to us to not have to deal with it all." The house had just gone on the market that day. I offered a full price offer plus bought the furniture. The deal was done!

Over the next year, my amazing house and my still agreed-upon divorce were a challenge. Looking back, I am honored by all the clients that hung in during that transition. A week after I moved in, there was a flood in the living room. After almost eight months of construction and trying to work and live around plumbing and power being shut off periodically; the clinic and my home were settled. The divorce finalized shortly after and the next level of learning how to care for my clients and myself was about to unfold.

CHAPTER

Five Holistic Components to Living in Comfort and Function

Life is a process, not a destination. Working together to support you in getting rid of your back pain and avoid surgery will be a process. My goal for you is a paradigm shift that feels so gentle you will be shocked at the new person you are at the end of this experience together.

We are going to walk through this process in five easy steps together. I will help you understand more about your body. We will work "with" your body instead of working "on" your body. I will also teach you how your environment plays into your journey back to health. What to do after to support your body so you maintain the progress you've made. And learn about complementary products and services that can enhance or speed up the process for you!

I deeply value working with Dr. Howard Cohn, of the Cohn Institute in Orange County, California. He has reminded me that finding your health is a journey not a destination. So many times we think, "If I do this, then I can do that." Yes and no. My guess is this is not the first resource you have tried to help with your back pain so far. You tried X and it didn't hold, which is why you have bought this book. Maybe you just need a new X. Right?

Or maybe you need a new paradigm of principles that will help you in a very gentle way find your Reverse Button back to your best comfort and function so you can avoid surgery and get back to living life fully and joyfully again!

Weaved through this whole book, the process and the stories, I encourage you to look for and feel for the principles that underlie all we are going to do together. My job is that of a facilitator or guide. Some like to call me a healer. I generally expand their definition of that word. I feel that my job, whether I am working directly with you or you are reading this book for support, is to set the environment for your body to find its best comfort and function. I do this through the following principles:

1. Self-Recognition

Self-recognition is half of what I do with people. So much of our culture is set up for us to disregard the messages our body is trying to communicate regularly. We numb out by use of TV, alcohol, drugs (legal and not), excess food, staying busy, and so on. I am just as excited when a client comes in and says, "I booked this appointment because last week I tripped in a hole in my yard and hurt my back; but now it is doing better." I am excited because they actually recognized the pain and that their body found its way back to its comfort and function. It found the Reverse Button! How many times do we hurt ourselves and think, "Suck it up, you are tough, just work through the pain"? While sometimes we are able to stuff and move forward, the problem is that it was stuffed and not released. So, the next time you go to pick up your socks off the floor or reach for a door knob and your back goes out; you are confused. I don't get it! I don't even have a reason for my back to go out. Yes, you do! And we will work together to help you find your self-recognition.

2. Meeting in the Right Relationship

It is important to me that we build trust with our health-care providers. Trust is earned when there is a mutual agreement of respect. I respect you are your own expert of your body. You have been in it longer than anyone else. I want to listen to what you have to say about it. Often-times clients will say, "I feel like somehow my back pain is connected to my knee but I don't know, the doctor says it is separate." I am the person to believe you. I want to work with your intelligence. With what you know about your body and with what we discover together. At your own rhythm of timing. I once asked an instructor, "How fast do you move the shoulder around?" He answered, "Not faster than you can listen." Before that, I had taken classes on energetic horse dancing. It is the ultimate give and take of energy in a beautiful flow of respect and meeting each other in right relationship. If either falls out of this balance, the dance ends.

3. Honoring What Arises

I tried to format this book in a way that is similar to how I work with clients individually. When a client comes in, I ask how their body is doing today. I listen carefully and make a plan of action based on my 1,500 hours of class time and seven years of experience. You might come in and tell me your back hurts and you are really worried about having to go in for surgery. I have you lay down on the table and the first thing I notice on an intuitive level is that the bones in your feet are bound up; so, I start my work there. You might be confused if this is your first time work-ing with a holistic practitioner. What I have learned is we honor what shows up first in our awareness. This book has structure and I trust you what you need the most or first will rise to the top for your understanding and healing first.

4. Going with the Flow
5. Less is More

These two principles go hand in hand. Once I've hon-ored what arose first, I go with the flow of what is next, and next, and so on. The man that developed Ortho-Bion-omy was a judo master and studied homeopathy. He said we need to go with the flow of nature to achieve more in the body and that we use the least amount of force to allow the body to rise up to do the most healing. By following the lead of your body to prioritize what needs to be released in what order, the ability to correct and hold happens quicker and is more complete.

6. Structure Governs Function

This is a saying originally from osteopathy, which is the roots of both Chiropractors and Ortho-Bionomists, and that we all can agree on. My take on this is just a little different. For chiropractors and osteopathic doctors, they are generally referring to your bones. If the bones are in a structure that looks like my skeleton in my office, then you are all good. I think of structure as a word that refers to so much more: structure of your nervous system, structure of your circulatory system, structure of your digestive system and so on. I think they each have structure as individual systems and also as a whole system together. I also think your full system has a structure in the universal system. All together finding structure in the whole system brings both comfort and function.

7. Going with Ease of Movements
8. Exaggerating the Patterns
9. Working "with" vs. Working "on"
10. Finding Comfort within Discomfort

I think these four all go together. As a facilitator of an environment for your body to find its best comfort and function, I am looking for, and teaching you to look for, the comfort within the discomfort. We often want to focus on what is not working and I am looking to remind the body of what does work. That is the trick to the Reverse Button. If I force your body (work "on" instead of "with") to move, then the body has a natural defense mechanism to not want to do that. Instead, I remind it gently, remember how good this position feels, I go with the ease of movement and exaggerate the comfort the body goes, "Awww, I was looking for the path back to that, thanks for reminding me," and will then make that be your most used path, or your super highway track. We found the Reverse Button together. Your body wants to work in comfort – it just got off track and needs the support to find its way back! We can do that together!

11. Being Present for Others without Judgment

This principle is so huge and can be challenging as a human being. Let's face it, as much as we don't want to, we judge a lot. We make decisions about people, books, and places in split seconds. My goal as we work together in the book or in person is that when we meet, we are both open and in present time. I will walk you through a self-care technique later in the book to help you navigate your world from being present. It is a true gift that I must stay conscious of at all times. I run the exercise I teach you through my mind probably twenty times a day to intentionally live the life I want to live. To be able to show up for my clients, my friends, and my family, in the respectful way I want to be with them. If you'd like a video of this exercise and other content not able to be put in the book, email me at: ReverseButtonBook@gmail.com with the subject line, "Bonus Content."

These principles I shared are a way of life and practiced will enhance your finding more comfort and function in all

CHAPTER

4

Your Body from a New Perspective

When I meet a new client to see if we are a good match, there are a lot of questions I go through. Some I learned in school and some that come up organically as the story unfolds. This process can take five to fifty minutes, depending on the person. Many clients note that I am not taking notes or typing into a computer like they have seen so many times with other healthcare providers. This is true for two reasons. One, I want to be fully engaged and listen to where you are at in this very moment. What your current priorities are. What I learned happens when we write in a chart, it can lock a person into that issue both in the client's and the practitioner's mind.

We are expecting there to still be the same problem; and when you go look for it I've learned the body is more than happy to recreate it for you. My goal is to meet you fresh each time and to let your story unfold in new ways and for your story to shift. You may forget all what you initially came in for. The body does this on purpose; my OBGYN told me that if it weren't for this amazing gift of the body to forget the pain, then we would never have a second child. The second reason I don't take notes is because while I am listening with my intellect and education to you and am forming a plan of action once the intake is over; I have to be ready to completely let go of my plan once I tune into your body. In Ortho-Bionomy, I was trained to feel from the physical to the energetic side of the body. To recognize what is yelling the loudest (the thing you most likely told me about in your intake), to the part of the body that is so busy holding everything together that you will never fully have comfort and function until it is addressed too.

I often explain to clients about Dr. Maria Montessori's brilliant work at the turn of the century, using observational science she discovered that until around age six we take in *everything* in our environment like a photograph – no filter! Around age six the filter, also known as the cognitive brain, starts sorting the information for us. This is the part of my brain I use to listen to your intake. The body is still taking in all the information though, just as before, with no filter. So, when I go to work with your body, I have to listen from my body to yours. Some call it intuition. Research has now shown there are more brain cells in the gut than the brain so the trendy phrase, is the "gut brain." I also like to explain that each of these "unfiltered photographs" can be thought of like train tracks. In one moment of time the flash went off and your body did its best job in that moment to make sure you didn't bleed to death; you didn't break a bone and that your eyes stayed level. Now to accomplish these three amazing feats your body did a lot of adjustments throughout (watch slow motion videos on people falling – it is amazing how the body can contort in a split second). It created one track in that moment. Every time we have a "trauma" – I use this word very loosely because it can be a physical or emotional trauma, it can be something small like stubbing your toe to something big like a death in the family – everything in between creates a track. What we do together will be to find your best track of comfort and function; and the best part is your body still has it in there! My job is to set up your environment for your body to find it and then make that be the super highway track that it goes to the most often!

If you were in my office, you would meet George. He/she is my skeleton and business partner that I can use as a visual of what I feel is going on with your body. (George is both a girl's and a boy's name in my family. So, when I got the skeleton my younger daughter asked if it was a boy or a girl. I said it was a George. She said, "OK" and the name stuck!) Something that is important to say here is when I am evaluating your body, I do not expect you will ever look exactly like George and neither should you. In the beginning of my Ortho training, I remember hearing that if a hunchbacked person comes into your office you do not try to make them straight backed like the skeleton. Your goal is to set up their body to find their best comfort and function. If you have seen someone with a lot of plastic surgery and they have tried to make their face perfectly symmetrical, it looks weird because it is not natural. We are not all supposed to look like George. We are each born unique and with our own best structure. This is also true with our individual neurological tracks that we have created in our bodies. They each have a purpose. They each should be honored for their contribution. Each track is a gift. Each track connects the whole body from the physical to the energetic.

Somehow our healthcare went down a path of specialization and looking at every complaint with the body as a separate issue. It is all connected! The hip bone's connected to the neck bone that is connected to the foot bone, and so on; sorry if I just got that song stuck in your head! I had a client that was in a hotel and she backed up and didn't realize how close the tub was behind her. She fell into the tub. When she came to see me, she complained about the pain in her back that happened from the fall. She didn't have a slow motion video taken of this fall. She had no idea of what all happened in that split second or what her body did to keep her alive. It was brilliant. It did its job. It created a new track to work from and was stuck there. When we started working together, the first thing I noticed was that her body still felt like it was falling. The energetic movement was still falling even though the physical body was sure they weren't anymore. I worked with the rhythm of the fall and gently rocked the body in the direction of the fall to remind it that yes you went in that direction. I then slightly exaggerated it and the body came back quickly and reset. It just needed a reminder that there was another option from where it was stuck at. If I would have only focused on the back pain, I could have moved bones and muscles around all day long; but it would not have held or would have needed an excessive amount of constant reminders before it may have even

Often at this point, I would put you on the table to see how things line up. Often a client will tell me very confidently that they have one leg shorter than the other. I confirm. I then lift their leg up, with a simple compression I set it back down and say, "And now you don't." I will be honest, it does not always work that way, every body is different, but often it does. I think this is a personal pet peeve of mine because of all the times I have been told this, shown images of this, and even been given shoe lifts two times. Your pelvis and your other horizontal planes, collar bone, sphenoid, and knees are all connected to your body trying to keep the eyes balanced; as well as being all connected to nearly everything else in both your physical and energetic body. Sometimes, and I have totally done this myself too, we are told something by someone in authority and we carry that as a fact, never to change, like one leg being longer than another. I encourage you to listen for the stories you are telling your body. Change is available. Other tracks are available.

Sometimes when I am working with a body, I will find a disconnection or a blockage in the information that needs to go through the nervous system or the fluids that need to go through the tubes of the body. I first really found this when working with a woman who trained dogs for a living.

I was working with her legs. It felt like bunched up balls of scar tissue throughout her legs. At first I was confused by what I felt. I know what cellulite feels like – which are toxins bunched up in the fat layer – but this was different. As we talked more, I realized that she had been bumped into roughly, repeatedly, by dogs for years. These bunching of cells were affecting the communication in her legs. Luckily we could work with the body to smooth that out!

After my last car accident where I was hit by a fully loaded log truck going fifty-five miles per hour in my Suburban that had stopped with traffic, I was in a lot of pain. Six months into my recovery, I was slipping backwards and the pain was increasing instead of decreasing. The osteopath I was working with had me in a shoe lift and was talking about a potential surgery. This was before I knew about Ortho-Bionomy, but just like you I was just open to try anything to avoid surgery and was open to trying anything to avoid the surgery. My older daughter was struggling with anxiety and depression at the time, and we were referred to an energetically gifted woman who also did work called EFT (Emotional Freedom Technique) and Bodytalk. I decided to make an appointment for myself, too. I was open to try anything to avoid the surgery – sound familiar? She worked with me and in one session I was better. I went back to the osteopath. He got all excited and asked, "Can I have her card? You won't need me again."

I was so confused. "But what did she do?" I asked.

He explained that when I was in the car accident, I was looping in my trauma and she helped me get on a different track so I didn't need to loop any more. I said, "But you were going to cut on me, and what about the shoe lift?"

He said, "You don't need them anymore."

I walked out of that office so confused and grateful that I avoided the surgery. It wasn't until I started to learn Ortho that I understood fully why this worked, she worked with my nervous system. She worked with my tracks! I will be forever grateful for that amazing woman!

While the pain from that car accident was gone, the original issues of my pelvis being unstable at times would pop up from time to time. It wasn't until about halfway through my Ortho training that I started to understand my pattern and started to see it enough in others I was working with to understand that *pain is communication in the body; so is instability*. This can be brought on by any of the tracks in the body. For me, my pelvis is my communicator. It tells me if I am either sorting through something emotional or trying to figure out how to relate to new information. Remember I said it is one of the horizontal planes. I now thank it for that information. I also get migraines still from time to time; I've learned they are to tell me when I'm taking on too much and not stopping to listen to my body. These are not easy communications to hear and many times I want to just "be tough" and "work through the pain" or numb it out and keep going. I've learned that is not to my benefit! Nor most of my clients.

I'm just as excited when a client recognizes their body's communication as I am when their pain is reduced! I have had two clients who processed their emotions primarily through talking, and we would rarely actually get to the table for work. They would return for appointment after appointment because their body recognized the release that was happening when we were together; long before they could recognize it for themselves. The exciting part is eventually they were able to recognize the releases! The "work" was happening for them!

All of this dance of listening is really about being in the right relationship with my clients and teaching them to be in the right relationship with their brilliant bodies. My goal when we work together is to help you find your best way to discover the most about yourself. Each of our timelines is unique. I have a family that comes in together all the time. They originally found me when I was working at the school, so they hold a belief the work can be very fast, so sometimes I even see all three of them in a regular appointment of thirty to forty-five minutes. I love working with them; because they find relief. They understand their tracks and the messages their bodies' are giving them.

With this newly gained perspective of your body, feel free to email me at: ReverseButtonBook@gmail.com with the subject: Additional Content to see some of the body charts and supporting documents I have referenced in this chapter.

CHAPTER

5

The Difference of Co-creative Work

know I've already said this before, but it lends its start to this chapter by saying it again. Every Practitioner is different, just like every body is different, and finding a great match feels amazing! At the Ortho Healing (OH) Center, the work I have developed in myself to share with you started back with Splash the horse, and learning to really listen deeply from a prey animal's energetic field that is so large they can feel you coming a long way away. If you haven't been introduced to the HeartMath Institute, look them up. They have the most amazing pictures of how large our energetic fields are and how they interact and when we are together. Horses are such great teachers of this because their organs are larger and so their energetic fields are larger.

Let's back up for a minute and talk about the word "energy." I know when I first was introduced to the word, I tried to skirt around it and would call it "magnetism," because somehow that seemed less woo-woo. But organizations like the HeartMath Institute have scientifically proven we all have an energetic field, just like we have a magnetic field. Heck, it was Einstein who said $E=MC^2$. The more comfortable I got with the word and that is just a fact, the more comfortable my clients were able to recognize the work that happened in the energetic field.

Just like in the last chapter, the whole body is connected throughout; so is the energetic field. I once saw a picture that made me so excited, I sent to my sister to print on her work printer and told her, "This is it – this is the visual that explains how the energetic field is connected." She shook her head at me and said, "I don't get it, but obviously you do!"

I did. I told her this image of lines all converging like a complicated spider's web was why I could work on her dog from hundreds of miles away. She once had called me and asked for me to come to her house seven hours away to work on her dog Hank. She was worried; he was so sick. I onomy, identified seven reflexes by name, and Advanced Instructor Sheri Covey brought their understanding to a practical application at the Rocky Mountain Ortho-Bionomy Center as the largest Ortho-Bionomy school in the world. The work of understanding the reflexes is growing exponentially through all that have worked with Sheri. My understanding, in this moment, is this is a universal language of vibrations that all beings can understand and can move easily through time and space within the energetic grid. There are thousands of reflexes. Arthur only named seven. And when I only focus on those seven, I miss hearing the rest. As I've opened my listening up, the language gets richer all the time. This is why my work has also been able to evolve to work with all beings from babies in utero, to 1,000-pound horses and everything in between. A perfect story for this section is about a beautiful, kind, soft-spoken, retired elementary school teacher in her sixties. She talked about many challenges with her body, but never talked about being concerned with the fact that her head shook uncontrollably at times. The reflexes were her answer to getting relief to something she never brought up because she didn't believe there was anything that could be done about it. When she would get quiet on the table, I could find the rhythm of the head shake and match that rhythm through her feet. It would loop over and over again. I would then take the matched rhythm in her feet and offer a slight exaggeration. It was just enough for her body to recognize another option and her head would settle.

Since Ortho-Bionomy is such a new modality in the state of Oregon, I have had to do a lot of community education. One of my favorite places to go is the Nautilus Gym in Oregon City. The ownership and I are very much in alignment of supporting the community in a variety of ways. They had invited me to an event to share my work. In front of a crowd of people, a woman with legs that looked like tree trunks lumbered up to the front. "Is there anything you can do for the swelling in my legs?" I'm not going to lie, this woman's body intimidated me, especially in front of a crowd of people. I put her on the table and started working just off her body offering her legs a rhythmic pumping action and a pattern arose. That pattern was a reflex, and by helping it taper through the dance it quieted to less, and less, until the flow in her legs had a whole new smooth flow like a constant stream. Someone in the crowd gasped, "Look at her legs!" They had dramatically changed. Two of the identified principles of Ortho-Bionomy are "going with the flow" and "less is more." That five- to ten-minute demonstration was all that woman needed for her body to find her Reverse Button and get back to her body's best comfort and function.

At a different community event, a woman came to my tent to try my work. I was offering five- to ten-minute free demonstrations. She told me she was dealing with pain throughout her body and was a diabetic. I worked with her feet because that was what rose for me intuitively as her highest priority. She left, and the next morning (it was a three-day event), she came back to the tent with friends, one after another nearly all day. She had woken up that morning and had the best numbers with her diabetes in years. Her body had found a Reverse Button that we weren't looking for directly, but it knew what the priority was and was not limited to what our beliefs in the moment were.

The body has an incredible desire and ability to heal itself. I belief this to the core. I also believe there is a time and space for us to use the medical options available to us. My goal with many of my clients is to avoid surgery; and often we do. Sometimes after working together though for a while we agree that it is time to seek medical intervention. Hospitals in Colorado have found that having Ortho-Bionomy post-surgery can speed recovery times about fifty percent. So far, the clients I have had that did need to go in for surgery we were actually able to speed recovery even faster than that. My favorite story is a client who went in for his four-week checkup and was sitting in the waiting room with people all in wheelchairs or walkers. He asked them when they had their surgery. All of them were all within a day of his. He had walked in by himself! When he saw the doctor, he was amazed. He had told him it would take at least twelve weeks with P.T. to be better. The doctor said he could release him now at the four-week mark. A second client had a very similar story: a month, not months to be better. This is the power of the work that I have been able to gather and offer through the Ortho Healing Center.

Now, I do have to be very honest that there are additional factors I need to share that help shape the work that happens through the Center. The first element is my business partner known as L.D. – some call him Little Dog, some Little Doctor, my favorite still is the Literary Dude. When I was at the Rocky Mountain Ortho-Bionomy Center I was honored enough to meet Brian and his dog Barry. Brian was blind and Barry was his business partner. My first time I really got what was happening between them was when we were in class and Sheri had to repeat a lesson to us twice on the same leg of the person on the table. Barry, who was an older, obese golden retriever, lumbered up with a humph sound and waddled through the crowd of people.

from when I was doing the energetic groundwork classes with the horses. I was told it was how all the birds in the sky knew to turn at the same time. It was nervous system to nervous systems reading off each other constantly through the energetic field. It was what animals do all the time. This was how L.D. was able to do what he did with clients. I started to notice that based on the work that was happening on the table, he would move around the room, supporting the client's nervous system by just being calm with them. It was giving their nervous system something to read off of. This why many of us have dogs. Coming home to that happiness just helps us be happy. When we are sad, our dogs are extra cuddly and know we are sad. No words are needed. They are reading us constantly. Clients started bringing me their dogs and booking appointments where I could work back and forth with the person and the dog, because often their health challenges would mirror each other. Then I had a regular client who started bringing her daughter and stopped booking for herself. I asked one day about it and she said, "Don't you know?"

"Know what?" I asked.

"I feel like I get a session just by sitting in the room with you when you work with my daughter. I don't need a separate session."

Of course it works human to human, too – we all have nervous systems. It still blew me away!

I have the best people that come to the clinic! One of those amazing people is an energetically gifted woman that has studied the metaphysical world for years and is fascinating to have conversations with. She came in for a session one day and I said, "Before we get started, I need to ask you a few questions that I think I'm ready for the answers to." I explained to her that when I work and clients ask questions, I generally hear the answer before they ever even finish asking the question. Often the answer comes in as a curt, exasperated, New York accent: my absolute alter internal voice. She smiled and said, "Yes, would you like to meet your guides?" I have seen gifted people for years for readings, but never once would I put myself into that category. I haven't been able to even get near the full English language equivalent to all that happens with source through me. What I can explain is that I know that my job, in co-creation with source and my guides, is to set up the environment for the body to do its best work and to listen and respond to the universal language that is being communicated. No matter what your beliefs are around this subject just trade out the words to something that feels comfortable for you to understand: God, Buddha, Universe, Goddess, etcetera. Again, I am still working on better words to explain what I experience. I do know, like I've said at the beginning of the chapter, all practitioners bring their gifts to their work and are different. This is my gift and I am deeply grateful to be sharing it with you. I was taught to be very careful about being called a "healer" because often ego will jump in and get in your way and will slow your work. What I do know deeply is I am a "facilitator." I set up environments for the body to do its best work with all resources available.

CHAPTER

6

Your Environment Matters

D
o you know how much your environment makes a difference in getting rid of your back pain? In the 1990s I was taught a word: ergonomics. I think this is what most people think about when I talk about your environment making a difference, but that is only a fraction of it. I was trained by the state of Oregon to be an ergonomics assessor. I went to my colleagues' workstations and made sure their computers were at the right level for their eyes and that the lumber support was actually supporting their backs. I made sure that their feet were sitting properly on the floor and their keyboards were at good angles for the wrists and shoulders. I have not worked in a traditional office setting in nearly twenty years, so I would hope this still goes on in some fashion today.

My clients all seem to have a general awareness around this concept. The challenge that comes for them, and me, too, is our "work" has become so portable that most of us don't just use a workstation, but work throughout the day from a phone, tablet, or laptop. I will be honest; I tried to set myself up for a marathon writing session for this book at my dining table, all factors above in consideration, and you know what happened? It slowed down my creative flow. I wrote slower than I do when I sit on my couch with my feet up, a pillow behind my back and fighting for the blanket with my dog. The ergonomic assessor in me is ashamed; but this is real life! This is what I know my clients are doing, and maybe you are doing right now as you are reading this!

I was in an Ortho class one day and the instructor shocked me to the core – she said that we didn't have to have perfect posture. We didn't have to stand up straight and force our backs into uncomfortable positions. I was so confused. I was told my whole life I needed to pay attention to that. Clients come in often with shame around not sitting up straight like they know they are "supposed to." Side note: whenever the words "supposed to" shows up, that is a waving red flag to me that usually means I need to really look at whatever it is I think I'm "supposed to" be doing and throw that idea right out the window. Ok, back to sitting up straight... this instructor said the body wants to be in comfort and function. When we force it to do anything that is uncomfortable, let alone painful, it will rebel like a teenager. We need to work with it, without force, to set up the environment for it to find its best comfort and function; this way it will want to remember how it got there.

So, why is sitting on the couch for me to write a good idea? Because I am consciously being aware of the environment I am setting up for my best comfort and function. I have favorite music playing softly in the background. I have a favorite blanket on my lap. My Hug Tea is brewed and sitting next to me. I have a vase of flowers set on the coffee table next to me. I have the lighting in the room soft but light enough I can see. I've given my body good nutrition and slept well. And, of course, my constant companion, L.D. is close too!

When I was working in the Montessori education world, I learned about the importance of setting the environment for the child to grow into their best self, not limited by the teacher (or they call them guides in Montessori speak). The guide takes the child through the environment. The environment needs to be created as so enticing that the child wants to do nothing else but be there because it satisfies something so deeply within them that they are drawn to it like a magnet. One of my favorite compliments at the clinic is when someone walks in and pauses and with a sigh will say, "Aww, it just feels good here." I beam with joy inside because I know we will have a good session. They have found a good match to bring their body to their best comfort and function. I had a Montessori teacher come in one day and she commented that even my dog water bowl was pretty. I said proudly, "Of course, I am still a Montessorian at heart!" Have you thought about what and who is in your environment? What makes you drawn in like a magnet and feel deeply met and satisfied on all levels of your consciousness?

Ortho-Bionomy was started by a British osteopath who also was into judo and homeopathy. One principle that carried over from osteopathy was "structure governs function." I love to debate the understanding of this principle. For many it means your bones need to be in place, like the bones on my skeleton George, and you will have good function. I look at this principle and go *very* broad with it. To me, I agree that your bones need to be in their best structure (not that they necessarily need to look like George), but so do your muscles, your fascia, your nerves, heck all the tubes of your body; and, yes, even your energetic body energy. I once heard the one-third rule and have loved it ever since. It says that you should have about one-third of the people in your life at a higher vibration than you; living the life you aspire to have. One-third of the people you spend time with should be at the same level as you, and one-third of the people you spend time with should be people that want to raise their vibration and you can give back to in some way. This is why I love working within groups for Ortho-Bionomy. I have attended Ortho classes and put on hundreds of demonstrations in group settings on the work that I do at the Center. The one-third rule generally shows up in any group that naturally comes together. Watch for it, it is fascinating that it was there all along. Coming together in a varied group gives our social nervous system several options to read off of. Remember your body has *so* many tracks, millions, billions, I don't know the exact number. *And* your body is constantly trying to be in its best comfort and function. For years I would try to figure out why in a group the work would amplify. I now know it is the power of all of us working together to find comfort and function together. We may all have different starting points but the goal is similar and that has power! Thanks to writing this book, the Reverse Button Programs were born to offer more group options regularly to my clients.

But, wait, what if you've been told your problems with your back are genetic? This doesn't really apply to you, does it? Yes, it still does! Thanks to the recent studies of epigenetics, we now know that we are not trapped by our genetics. They are tracks in our bodies that were passed through our heritage, but they are not necessarily tracks that have to be activated. By putting ourselves in intentional environments that focus on living our best comfort and function the most amazing things can happen.

One of my favorite stories about the power of the body to heal was a client who came in with a torn muscle in her arm. She couldn't lift her arm away from her body; it just hung limp. She had seen a doctor who confirmed the tear, and she was told it would just take a couple of months to heal. To measure the tear, I laid my fingers next to it. It was six fingers long and the depth was as deep as my first knuckle that could go into the gap. We set to work together, L.D. laying under the table for support. I asked her to close her eyes and tell me about a happy color. She picked her color. Then I told her we were going to build a bridge over this gap in her arm. I asked her many questions to take her to this happy place building her bridge out of whatever material she wanted, during an ideal day for her and so on. We continued until the tissue filled in and my fingers were pushed out of the gap. It took about twenty minutes. I asked her to raise her arm when we were done. It worked! We had created a pleasant environment in imagination that stimulated all the happy rebuilding cells in her body. And because we were laying it down board by board with structure there was no bunching of the cells like what happens when the body creates scar tissue. When people challenge me on this concept, I tell them to think about this … you get a cut and the body floods the cut with blood to rebuild as quickly as possible to keep you from bleeding to death. We are calling on that same function in the body and adding structure and guidance at the same time. A colleague in Portland, Rosi Goldsmith, first introduced this concept to me blending meditation and Ortho together. She had been working on a study with a medical doctor on feet to have published.

Along similar lines with using meditation and Ortho together, my practice expanded to being able to offer remote sessions. In a previous chapter I talked about working with my sister's dog Hank. Later I explored it with a blind client of mine. While she was extremely capable of getting herself around the city using public transportation, it was an extreme effort for her to make it to my office. Then once there, we could only work about fifteen minutes together before her body had enough. When one sense is challenged, often the other senses will be heightened to compensate. I offered a remote session. I would text her when I started and when I finished and then we would compare notes. During that time, I would be in my office using my imagination, as if her body was in front of me, and could feel her through the energy matrix just the same. We were able to move up to thirty minutes of work for her body! Then I met a woman who lived in California that wanted to work with me. I told her that I was able to work remotely and we ended up evolving together even further by having her stay on the phone with me, and for me to talk with her just the same as she was in the clinic. To date, I think the remote sessions may be some of my favorites because they are not confined by three dimensions.

Ortho-Bionomy had a wave of massage therapists that came to the work about twenty to thirty years ago that made a big impact on the way many practice this work. People sign up for a certain amount of time to be touched and lay on a table. I've been told that when Arthur worked with people, they would be sitting, standing, and laying down over a twenty-minute period, and then he would walk with them for about twenty minutes. I was fascinated with this concept. I started playing with vertical work. One of the first people I tried it with was a friend in my living room. I told her that since she didn't have a table to stop her, she could move in any direction she felt she needed to. I started bringing in reflexive compressions into her back and she started to turn her feet, before I knew it, she pirouetted out of my living room into my kitchen, paused, and then pirouetted back. I stood there with my jaw dropped. She said, "Was that OK? You said I could move my feet."

"Of course," I said, "I just didn't know that could happen. How do you feel?"

She said, "Amazing! I feel like I am no longer holding my son."

I asked her to explain more and she said she had a high-needs child over twenty years ago that was very difficult to carry, and energetically she had been carrying him for all those years. She felt that she was free from that weight and body contortion she had been doing for twenty years! I was in love with vertical work from then on out!

What if you can't move around and you aren't so sure about the remote sessions? Good news – I have had clients stay in their scooters or sit in chairs. Even without direct access to their back, we can accomplish a lot of work to support their back through working with their extremities and offering cranial Ortho. Now before being exposed to Ortho, my favorite modality was cranialsacral work. I loved how gentle yet profound it would feel in my whole body. Actually, the first time I received an Ortho session that was how I would describe it to others. I would say, "It's like cranialsacral for the whole body, gentle and yet profound!" In school, I was able to meet people who were trained in both and asked what they thought the difference was, because after my first Ortho cranial, I felt the bones in my face working on realignment for a month. It was the craziest, coolest experience ever! It was explained to me that craniosacral is working through a series of waves that are going through the body, which is amazing and cool. With cranial Ortho, to me, we are tracking so much more; from the physical to the energetic and listening for the universal language of the reflexes along the way. So, for one of my clients who is in a scooter, this is my favorite thing to do with him. His whole body benefits and profound work happens!

One day I was working at a barn on a very special horse named Bacardi. He ended up not needing the full hour I was booked for, so I offered his owner a little vertical work in the barn. She had a back-fusion surgery many years before and still had issues with back pain regularly. Her back didn't move with ease or function. I took the last ten minutes and worked with her. She paid and I left. She contacted me shortly after for a full appointment for herself. She couldn't believe in such a short amount of time that she had received such a tremendous amount of relief. I may have only touched her for ten minutes, but she had also been in the same space while I was working with her horse for the fifty minutes beforehand. Her body was responding to it all!

Animals are such a tremendous gift within our environments. Not only is it helpful for L.D. to lay down in the room and be mellow so your nervous system can be reminded on how being mellow together works, he has learned to track through a body with me.

I talked about the gift of our animals in the previous chapter. I used to joke that when I widow, I would become a crazy dog lady because my husband had said he was allergic and couldn't have a dog. Then one day he visited his sister and she was dating a guy with an Australian Shepherd. All the pictures of the trip had him and this dog hanging out. My daughters commented immediately! "What happened to your allergy?" He said that he didn't know there were cool dogs out there. Shortly after that, he was hunting with my sister's husband. There had been mini Australian Shepherds on the hunt and when he came home, he said, "Did you know they make those dogs in boat size!"

I said, "What?"

He said, "You know, the cool dogs in a size that would fit well on my boat! I think we should look at getting a two-year-old."

I couldn't believe my ears! I jumped on it right away! At the time, my sister's friend had just had puppies and asked us over to help socialize them. They were all sold, so I thought it was safe. Well, I fell in love with the runt, and as he was cuddled in my neck under my hair, I was told his sale fell through and they were looking for a home for him. It was set! We picked each other. Little did I know that his presence would change the whole environment of our house. My husband who never could leave his work frustrations at work suddenly was greeted by the happiest, loving creature that just wanted his attention and to play with him. It changed our house forever. It changed my husband forever. I now think if he had more time, he would be the crazy dog guy because they have been so good to have in his life. Later we did end up rescuing an older mini cattle dog and when we divorced a couple of years later neither of us really wanted to give either dog up. Eventually one dog loved the country and the other the city, so, ultimately, they decided. But we both had a dog for our new homes and I am forever grateful that these loving energies greet us every day and offer cuddles every night!

CHAPTER

Health Maintenance Empowerment

At the end of a session, if you are on a table, I'll have you roll to your side and push yourself up slowly. Even though the work can feel so gentle and relaxing, it can be really profound to be relating to everything in your environment and body from a perspective it had forgotten about for a while, and sometimes it's been a very long while. I ask clients to sit for a few minutes so their body can get used to being upright again and drink some water. Often the body feels dehydrated at the end of the session. It truly is amazing how much is happening in there. I had one client, who was a macho, six-and-a-half-foot guy, try to jump off my table (I know he was thinking, yeah, that wasn't much of anything). He lost his balance, hit the wall, and was forced to sit back down. He looked at me in shock. I said, "Yes, your body just went through a lot; let's give it a moment to find itself again!" I will then invite clients to take a couple of laps around the table to give their bodies a chance to integrate. Bilateral movement, whether it is walking or swimming, is really helpful for the body to recognize the track that it currently is on and to bring all aspects from the physical and the energetic up to speed! Occasionally some will comment they feel high or altered and not sure if they can drive. For those clients, I offer brain gym support: their left and right brains are forgetting how to collaborate together. I have them do prayer hands and gently move back and forth across their midline, starting in the middle and slowly working their way above their head as far as they can go without hurting their shoulders. It always makes me think of a beautiful dance from India. At the top I have them take a big breath. I never make it to the top without a big yawn, which is a brilliant release, too. They slowly let their fingers wiggle back down to their sides and take another lap around my table in each direction, and they generally feel centered and able to drive.

I explain to clients what is considered normal post-session experiences:

1. They get off the table and it's a miracle and their pain is gone! We love it when that happens!

2. They get off the table and they feel nice and relaxed. A gradual correction happens. Over the next several days they may notice odd sensations throughout their body as the body pings the information through the nervous system trying to make sure this is really the best comfort and function option before settling on its choice.

3. They get off the table and are nice and relaxed. They pay me and leave and think that was a big waste of time and money. Then three days later they go to reach for their socks and there is no pain – what! It was nothing, nothing, nothing … better!

All nervous systems and issues are different. I can't tell you which you will experience. I know that most work for me gradually corrects over a couple of days. Most of the time, post session looks like this for me: I can barely get off the table because my pelvis likes to make sure it is boss, and until it decides on how it wants to relate to the Reverse Button that was just found, it feels a bit cranky and stiff. Then I will shake violently (we will talk more about this in the next chapter) for about twenty minutes. I am freezing cold to the core! The next day it's sunshine and roses! I've learned to trust this rhythm in my body and each of my clients finds theirs, too.

After the first session, I like to have a client come back in seven to ten days. I give them the homework of paying attention to their bodies. I think this is big homework for at least half of my clients who have been training to survive by ignoring all messages from the body. I tell them when they come back, I am going to want to know:

- What happened in the first three days? Were they able to find any comfort and function?
- What happened in the three or more days after? Did it hold? If so, how long?

This information helps me decide where to go next. If they say, "Yes I found comfort and it lasted about a week and then I lost it," I know we are on the right track and we just need to reinforce the work we did last time. If they say, "It was slightly better and still is," then I know we have a part of it, but there are more parts of the body that need to be brought into consideration for full comfort and function to be achieved. If they say, "Never found any comfort," I know I need to dig deeper in my tool bag. Luckily I have over 10,000 hours collectively between classes, life experiences and seven years in my practice so far. We simply need to take a different approach.

One tool I love to do with clients and to share with them as a self-care post session is called running dimensions and learning to be very present. When a client continues to have problems that are all on one side of the body, this is a good tool. When I work with someone who is constantly talking about the accident they were in and their story doesn't progress as we work together, I will use this tool.

For me, this tool came into play when I realized I had been rear-ended three times and had no awareness of my back energy at all. I have my client stand and face me. I then have them close their eyes (this is something you can do alone and even better with a friend. I do this probably ten to twenty times a day – you get faster once you learn it and can run it in your mind's eye. When you do this with another person though it does amplify the work!). Next, I ask them to tell me what do they notice first, no judgments, their head or feet? Whichever they noticed first, I then have them repeat a reflexive statement with me. They can either physically move their body with it, or just in their mind's eye. The pattern goes, "Here is your preference, here is your preference, here is your preference, hold." In the stillness of the hold, I encourage them to let their body unwind and move any direction that it needs to do. We are standing so they have full freedom of movement. Some have big movements; some have very little movement. I tell them to let it go as long as it wants. If you feel stuck or that you are looping in the same pattern, go ahead and repeat the words again. Move until it tapers into a quiet infinity. Then open your eyes. Recheck. Do you still notice your head of feet more or do they feel more balanced. If they are not balanced I have them repeat the whole process again. Generally, by the second time they feel more balanced. If not, I tell them that is OK; let's go to the next dimension and see if something there needs to shift first. The next dimension is side to side. Which do you notice first or can go toward with more ease? Choose that side and repeat the reflexive words just like before, "here's your preference, here's your preference, here's your preference, hold." Follow this all the way through just as before. Next is front to back. If you are standing belly to belly, you might want to step to one side so you don't blast the other person. Run your dimensions again. "Here's your preference, here's your preference, here's your preference, hold." When you feel you have achieved balance in all three dimensions, then I tell you that I was taught the top/bottom or head/toe is your relationship with the universal and the earth. The side to side is your relationship to self. And the front/back is your relationship to the future and past. For many, this explanation helps them find a clearer picture of why they have been struggling with their pain and can release a lot! It is a powerful tool!

For me, this is when I realized I didn't have any recognition of my back energetically. I did this exercise many times before I could ever get the front and back to balance. The first time I did this in a class with a partner, the instructor walked around us while we had our eyes closed. It freaked me out because I could not feel my partner when she walked behind me. It was blank. No sensation at all! Then we ran our dimensions and slowly over time I could feel it. When I reflected on this, I knew immediately this is why I had been rear-ended three times. I didn't want to deal with my past at all! And even though I had spent years in therapy trying to talk through everything, it just neurologically reinforced the trauma of my past and I didn't want to go there. Since I have learned this skill, I play with it all the time! To do my work effectively with clients, I need to stay in present time and be present for them. I run it before a session, sometimes several times during a session and after a session to clear myself. If I don't then odd issues come up in my life that sometimes take me a bit to realize aren't mine; they are a client's that I didn't clear from

Everyone's healing journey is different. Sometimes the healing journey isn't as kind or pleasant as we want to believe it should be. If you have ever detoxed, you know what I mean. When trying to get toxins out of your body, you will feel like you are getting the flu for a couple of days. You may ooze stink from your pores. Your bathroom time may clear the house. Have gratitude: your body is working toward its comfort and function. For me, I love journaling to track this journey. It helps keep me honest of how I feel in the moment and how it changes. Whenever I work with someone's organs, I always tell them, "Now, you may have a cleanse-like effect from this work. When you are running to the bathroom for the tenth time for the day, remember to say, "Yeah, body!" Not "What the heck did Abby do?"" It always makes them smile and often they thank me the next time I see them for the warning. We need to say, "Yeah, body!" daily! I know you have real pain and you also have an amazing amount of things that are working well in your body every day. Remember to celebrate them too. What we tell ourselves our body is listening to: Be kind! Be loving! Celebrate what is working!

What if we do absolutely everything together and we still have to have a surgery. Did we fail? Trust me, I recently had to have a biopsy. My first time ever being violated by being cut on. I chose it; but it brought me a whole new passion and compassion for my clients. It is my absolute goal to help keep you from a surgery. But if it does come to that; know and trust the strengthening we have done together for your nervous system before and the post-surgical plan we will have in place will get you back on your feet faster than any doctor will believe! I know I shared a bit in a previous chapter about Colorado hospitals finding about fifty percent faster recovery post-surgical with Ortho-Bionomy. So far, I have found recovery only taking about one-third the time out of my clinic!

The goal is to avoid surgery whenever possible. So far, my favorite story is of a vibrant, beautiful woman, who surprises everyone when she says she is a grandmother. As I age, I know grandparents are getting younger looking all the time; especially since many people I went to high school with are now grandparents. Anyway, back to her awesome story. We had been working together for several years now. When I first met her, she was confident she was needing surgery for her knees. She had issues with pain in her back and feet. She taught Zumba and sometimes other exercise classes throughout the week. She was fit and healthy, but the knees were taking the brunt of the activity. To date, we see each other about every two weeks for about twenty to thirty minutes of work. When she dances, she does wear a neoprene compression sleeve for added support – I told her to think it is me gently holding her knee in place and keeping it reminded of its best comfort and function! She uses mud from the Dead Sea that I recommended and Molecular Hydrogen for added support. We will talk more about those in the next chapter. The key is that together we have averted a surgery for years now that she thought was the only option when I first met her.

About a week ago, I was sharing Zumba Grandma's story with a new client, and she stopped me and said, "Wait, you could help me avoid a surgery?" I said yes! She had been in to see me for swelling in her foot which was better; so that day we focused on her knee. As we worked though her knee, her digestion showed up as an issue (often knees and digestion show up together). I followed that up to right shoulder and upper back. Down her arm to a place on her wrist. As soon as the wrist released, her tummy started to gurgle. This was a sign that the body is in rest and digest! I was so excited! She got off the table and started on her laps, and she had the biggest grin on her face – "I have no pain," she said. "I have no pain!" Her arms went above her head and she took a victory lap like she was in a Rocky movie! We hugged and celebrated together.

Other questions I get often is what about physical exercise to do post-session? Should I take it easy? Go work out? Do you have anything specific? As I said above, sometimes I recommend a self-care technique that will help strengthen the neurological pathway. Especially if I think you are someone who has a strong repetitive option in your life that we will be fighting against to keep this better functioning track to hold. So here is my best advice: if you are a runner, then run. If you have never run before, let's see how your body does before we try something new. I want you to leave my office and live your life. You are meant to move and one of the biggest challenges in our current life is being sedentary. Now if you get home from your session and you think, wow, I need a nap – listen to that if at all possible. Your body restores while you are asleep. I once slept for fourteen hours after receiving a session from my Ortho-Bionomy mentor, Sheri Covey; profound healing happened that day! When we sleep, our body is doing big work and is telling you to get out of the way so it can finish! Sometimes people will tell me they will have a burst of energy and need to go for a walk. Again, honor that! The bilateral movement will help your body reorganize around this track much faster. And remember at the beginning of this book I talked about research regarding longevity that says you need three things to live well into your later years: community (social nervous system support), science-based nutrition (we'll talk about that soon) and walking as the best exercise! Now I love yoga and Zumba and really dancing of any kind. So live life; but I won't be the one to tell you exactly what exercise you should or should not do. If it feels good and makes you and your body happy – I would continue with that one and do it daily! And if your body is struggling to keep up with something you love; let's make sure we find your Reverse Button so you can have that option in your life as long as possible! If you'd like some additional videos or quick reference sheets about this chapter email me at: ReverseButtonBook@gmail.com with the subject: "Additional Content".

Holistic Support – Mind, Body, and Spirit

've learned a lot about a lot of things from the wide variety of classes at the clinic to help my community live well holistically: from the food they consume, to how clean their home chemical free, to products to support their bodies post session. We've already talked about environment, now let's dive a little deeper into what else can support you to living in your best comfort and function – pain free!

I hosted a retreat weekend around this book during the final stages of the writing process, and a lovely couple from Texas came to participate. In their final interview they shared they were really surprised about the food. They figured as a health retreat to help them get rid of their back pain they would be fed only "rabbit food"; but she had eaten well and it all tasted good, too! This same woman said that every time she went to the doctor to talk about anything from her back pain to her bunion the doctor would tell her she just needed to lose weight. After the Reverse Button Retreat, she learned that she could accomplish that in many ways. I shared about an easy, plant based nutritional support system that I used to get rid of my post-divorce weight and now use to maintain my overall health. I taught the group about the importance of eating whole foods, and drinking half your body weight in ounces of water a day (example if you weigh 200 pounds, you should drink at least 100 ounces of water a day).

At the retreat, we also talked about how you can eat absolutely perfectly and still gain weight without your nervous system being supported. The group shared their frustrations with how weight and back pain seemed to go hand-in-hand. I told the story of a client who had been seeing me for years for back and knee pain. Her lower half of her body was constantly swollen with fluid and my primary job was to help move the fluid for her. While the bodywork had helped keep her functioning, when we started adding post products that I offer at that clinic, her function really began to change. First, she started putting mud from the Dead Sea on her knees. She is a dog trainer and agility judge so she is on her feet and needs to be able to move around. The mud was helping! The Dead Sea is the lowest point on Earth. Five rivers flow in and nothing comes out except through evaporation, so the minerals have been concentrating there for thousands of years. Historical figures have written about the therapeutic and beauty qualities. Cleopatra was said to ride, by camel, four months of every year to go spread the mud on her body and lay in the waters. Today nearly two million people a year go to the Dead Sea to put the mud on their bodies and to soak in the water for inflammation reduction, skin conditions, and so much more.

After seeing results with the bodywork and mud combination, she decided to go ahead and try the Weightloss Made Simple Plan I offer to reduce weight next. She will tell you that she is a skeptic on many levels and pretty set in her mind about what foods she likes and doesn't like. Just like my client from Texas who said she believed that all meals needed to have bread before the retreat weekend. When the dog trainer decided to do the Simple Plan, she didn't tell me at first because she had access to through the clinic directly online. She just came in for a session and the fluid on her legs was gone. I asked what she had done different. She said she was using the Simple Plan with the molecular hydrogen and alkalinity support products. I was blown away! Systematically her inflammation was down for her whole body! Between getting the minerals from the Dead Sea through her skin and now the Alkalinity and the Hydrogen inside of her, the bodywork we were doing together was able to hold longer! It was incredible! She came back a couple weeks later and said it happened for her sister too! Her sister lived in Iowa and had been having regular bodywork for her similar inflammation issues and she started on the same products and the massage therapist was just baffled that there was no excess of fluid to move, as she had done for so many years for her before that.

In the retreat we talked about how sometimes you just don't know where to start with making a shift in your food. Fad diets come and go. One month fats are good the next they are bad, it's enough to drive us all crazy. I love Dr. Howard Cohn, who said, "Health is not an event, it's a lifestyle." I think this is *so* important to set your mindset around. Yo-yo dieting is not helpful for anyone's health. Finding what works for you and setting a routine you can stick with is paramount. I love Dr. Cohn also says, "No one chased you down and shoved the doughnut in your mouth."

What food goes into our mouth is something we have complete control over, if we bring it into our consciousness. Don't get me wrong, I do recognize the struggle of being an emotional eater – I am right there with you, but Mrs. Texas's doctor was partially right: if we want to live without back pain then we do need to get our weight under control too. We will have better function. My general rule of thumb that I learned from my daughter's first grade teacher that has served our family well for years is this: nothing with more than ten grams of sugar, no artificial colors, or preservatives, and all the ingredients need to be something you can actually imagine growing somewhere. In my family I taught my kids at a very young age to read labels and think about what they are putting in the bodies. Now we are not perfect and each of us has gone on our own journey with this; but stop and think about the logic here and it makes sense. Real food equals real fuel. Food is fuel, minerals are building blocks we need. It is our job to give our body what it needs to have its best comfort and function and while the doughnut may feel good emotionally for a few minutes, an hour later it does not, years later stacked in your body … it does not.

For me, there was a chapter of my life when I was between careers and absolutely loved to cook and garden and had lots of time to prepare healthy food for myself and my family. And then there is the chapter in now where a towel hangs in my kitchen that reads: I only have a kitchen because it came with the house. I have found an amazing personal chef. She does my grocery shopping, plans my meals, keeps my diet way more varied than I ever did, provides me fresh, local, organic when possible foods. If you come to my house, we lovingly just call it, "Sarah food." She is a tremendous gift in my life. And best part: it saves me money! Yep, I learned that I wasted a lot of money buying extra food that got thrown out every week. I wasted a lot of time and energy with prepping, cooking, and clean up that I can now devote to other activities I want to do. If you are reading this and say, that is nice for you Abby but the Red Hare Catering won't deliver where I live. I say, look online; now more than ever we have healthy options that can be delivered to our doors to work with our busy, fast-paced lives. No excuses ladies. I often hear – eating well is too expensive, too time consuming, etc. Not being able to move because your back pain is so bad is expensive and time consuming. This is a mind-shift. A decision. And that can happen in this very moment you are reading this book. Decide you are worth the investment in your health. Decide you are going be mindful of the fuel you put in your body because you want to live well into your second half of life! I learned a new term recently: "playspan." I love this. I talked earlier that experts are saying for longevity you need: community, science-based nutrition, and exercise (ideally walking). These are the building blocks to help us live longer, but don't you want to live well, not just longer? "Playspan" is increasing your quality of life so you can play well into your second half of life!

OK, a few more words on food because it really is a huge topic. This book is not about weight loss, but if I can help you think about your food a little different, then perhaps I can help send you down the path to better back health that we are striving for in this book. At one point in my life I had to take very high doses of iron to keep me from having seizures. My liver protested greatly and swelled up so it stuck out from under my ribs. First, I learned about the importance of regular detoxing for the body to help flush out toxins. We have two systems for this: the skin and the organs. To support both, I eat moringa (a superfood plant) every day which has reduced my need for traditional iron supplements. One to two times a month I drink a moringa-and-seneca tea to flush anything stuck in my digestive track. If you have never drank anything like this before, just make sure that you really listen to your body and get up and go to the bathroom as soon as you start to notice an urge to go. I always give clients this warning and half the time they come back and say, "oh, that was no big deal" and the other half come back and say, "oh my gosh, I am so glad you warned me that was *very* effective and cleaned me out!" I also detox weekly through my skin to give my organs a break. Many years ago, a naturopath had me start with foot baths, a simple tub (I actually used my stock pot for quite a while before I went to the Dollar Tree and bought a dish tub) and Epsom salts. Later I learned that Epsom Salt is primarily just magnesium. The Dead Sea Salts are a higher concentration of magnesium plus twenty-five other minerals put together in perfect harmony, so I switched! I tell clients, it's like you can take a vitamin C tablet or eat the whole orange … the body needs the brilliance that nature put together in the whole orange – use the Dead Sea Mud and/or Salts! I then moved to a house with a claw-foot tub, my first tub I could fully submerge my body into. Now, weekly I spread a thin layer of Dead Sea mud over my whole body as my tub fills. I then sprinkle about a tablespoon of Dead Sea Salt into my bath water and get in and soak for twenty to thirty minutes. It is my mind, body, soul reset each week. If something comes up and I can't get to my tub, I will still do a foot soak and if life is really crazy or I am traveling, I will put the mud on under my clothes. I am committed to detoxing regularly, supporting my organs and keeping my skin healthy. It all matters!

So good and bad news, you can do all the things with your food I was talking about and still end up acid in your body – why? Because you either microwaved your food, you ate it fast, or you were thinking not-so-good thoughts while you were eating your perfect meal. So, what can we do about that? Many know the concept that bad things can't grow in an alkaline state, so the more we can be there the better for longevity and "playspan." Dr. Cohn tells an awesome story about how he just got tired of people lying to him in his office. He would tell them that eating inflammatory foods like gluten, dairy, sugar, eggs, etcetera were harming their body and they would say OK, I won't, and then they do. We are human! We are social beings and we have our life around social foods. I am a total foodie – I get it! So, I was extra excited to find that Dr. Cohn put together a simple capsule of natural ingredients that could be a "hall pass" for the day's activities. I say this with the caveat that I still think you should try to give your body good fuel, but in case you are human like the rest of us and eat your good food choices on the go in a stressed state, then know there is an option to balance out the damage you did during the day while you sleep! A few of my clients take this during the day and have been able to get off their prescription drugs for acid reduction, (insert legal disclaimer here – while it is your body and you know your body better than anyone else, legally I need to say – always consult with your doctor). The idea of this "hall pass" is you can vary your amount you take based on how "acidic you were for the day." For example in general I take two to four at night before bed. When I went to Mexico for my sister's fortieth birthday to an all-inclusive resort, I took eight at night! And I woke up each day feeling amazing, no food or drink hangover! Supposedly this has become quite a popular product in colleges: "How many boosters did you need to get to class this morning?" I dose myself through muscle testing and teach my clients how to do the same for them.

As a clinic owner, I have sales reps come by regularly trying to sell me new options for the clinic. I had one who tried to sell me a very expensive water filter system. She told me that the body doesn't utilize acidic water, only alkaline water. That is why you can sometimes feel dehydrated, even though you drank a lot of water that day. She set up her testing kit and showed me different water samples she had brought with her. I then asked if we could test the water in my house. Tap water was acidic. But interestingly enough, the water in my Brita countertop filter and my filtered fridge water both were neutral like her expensive filter was going to offer me. Next came a guy with a tester that would tell you how much oxidation you were getting in your blood. He had me put my hand on his machine and as it was calculating he said that most of us don't get enough green vegetables in our lives to bring the blood health to where it needed to be. He told me that clinics can charge for a test, then put clients on his vitamins to fix it and then charge for the follow up test to prove they worked. As he was talking my numbers kept rising. He looked up at me and said, "I've never seen anyone's numbers be this high before." I confirmed, "Even after you have people take your supplements?" He said yes. I just smiled. I said, "Yes, I have an awesome, simple program at my clinic that helps clients balance their alkalinity through plant based products." He left without a sale.

Not all my clients use all products I have at my clinic. Some decide that they will just start with one post-support product and even that has shown incredible results. I had a woman who came in for a detached ligament that had wrapped around her ankle. She saw me for a few Ortho sessions and usually a ligament tear can repair in one to two sessions so I was baffled that she wasn't better in four sessions. I sent her in for an MRI. The doctors came back that she needed surgery because the ligament had wrapped itself around her ankle. She called me panicked. She was a single mom with three jobs. She did not have time for this. She was just carrying a load of laundry upstairs and tripped, this is crazy! I told her I would talk with my mentor in Ortho-Bionomy and see if she had any suggestions. Her suggestion: make a post-surgical plan and help this woman get back on her feet as soon as possible. I called the client back and she still said, "No, Abby, you have to help me!" I said, "OK, I let's try this. Call the surgeon and make the appointment. It will take some time to get in. In the meantime, let's put Dead Sea Mud, a plastic bag, and a sock on your foot and let's see where we can get with that in conjunction with the Ortho." She agreed. She took a picture of her fat ankle that night, and then again the next morning. It looked normal! She called me and said it still hurt, so she came in for a thirty-minute session and we realigned the bones in her foot. She did two more mud treatments and was back to fully running the next week. *No surgery!*

Another client who just uses the Dead Sea Mud and Skin Care Products in conjunction with her bodywork at the clinic has had incredible shifts in her overall health. She had been seeing me for several years to help her body stay functioning. As a chef she is on her feet for long periods of time. As a woman she had spent twenty years with fertility drugs in her body trying to have a baby. When she first came to the clinic she said, "I walk like a China doll." She took the tiniest steps because her pelvis was so locked up. With regular sessions we were able to bring functionality in to her movements again. Then about two years ago she started using mud to detox and switched many of her skin care regimen to include products that had the Dead Sea Minerals in them too. Her appointments started spreading out because the minerals were helping her hold the work longer in her body. Then one day at an Open House event at the clinic, she was sitting around a table with several women, eating a piece of cheesecake and she told them she had lost about fifteen pounds because of the Dead Sea products. She said she hadn't been able to lose weight in many, many years and that the only thing she had changed was adding those products in. She took another bite of cheesecake, and said, "And obviously, I haven't changed my eating habits." I was blown away. As time went on and she kept losing, we talked about it and how much had been stuck in her body with all the years of fertility drugs and we believe the mud and minerals of the Dead Sea have been able to help her finally release them!

Another favorite post-care product we have at the clinic is the molecular hydrogen called Recovery. If someone wants help with inflammation, quick and easy as a tablet, this is perfect for them. In the same day, I had a client call, panicked. He had seen me a few weeks before because he thought he was ready for surgery and a friend suggested he come see me first. He had a session and I recommended Recovery and Mud Therapy Foot Cream for him as a post-care plan because he didn't want to deal with the messiness of the mud. Side note: clients have reported the foot cream as the best first aid cream that is good for just about everything from sore muscles, to cold sores, to burns, to hemorrhoids. He called that day because he had to drive all day for work and he had run out of Recovery and really thought our trifecta of Ortho, Recovery and Foot Cream was working for him. I told him I had a shipment coming in that day by eight p.m. He asked if I had any in my personal stash; I could give him just to get by for the day. I said yes, and he swung by the clinic before work and promised to be back that night to pick up more bottles. My first client then walked in for the day in the middle of a full-blown migraine and my heart went out to her. For years when she would get one, she would come into the clinic and I could help her calm her body down so it wasn't as bad. With the

Recovery though she had been keeping them at bay; so, I asked what happened. What changed? She said, she had run out of Recovery. I told her that I had a shipment coming in that night and she said, "Good, I'll send my husband over when it comes in." I gave her my last tablet that I had personally for her post-support for the day.

At times I will recommend regularly to clients to use homeopathy, like arnica for physical and emotional bruising. Often, I will share stories about high quality essential oils being used for health support to cleaning your house. I clean the whole clinic with silver-threaded microfiber cloths and oils. When I had a hot tub, I ran it on geranium oil instead of chemicals. What I have learned in oil classes is that you can put an oil on the bottom of your foot and it can be tested in the mouth within seconds. It really made me stop and think about our largest organ: our skin and just how important it is to take care of it and to stop and think about what we put on it because that will be absorbed in quickly!

So, what about exercise for post care? I get this question a lot. I do teach self-care for the back and we've talked about those in a different chapter. I've talked about the longevity study about the importance of walking and I highly agree that bi-lateral movement is extremely important for the whole of the body to work together in a holistic way. But this sometimes surprises people when I say, my belief around exercise is it is movement that needs to be daily and ideally something that brings you joy! So, dance like no one is watching! Crank up the tunes while you make dinner! Find a fun class that excites you like Zumba or whatever gets you going. For a time period in Oregon the weather is not so great and I am a fair-weather walker, so I looked at what I can do. I have three flights of stairs in my house. What if, at minimum I take a few minutes while I wait for my kettle to boil again for tea to do at least ten flights of stairs together? I evolved this to add different arm movements, stretches at the top of the stairs and fun music. I did try to include my dog who thought it was so much fun for about two days. Then I had to resort to putting him a on a leash to keep up with me. Then on day four, on the fourth trip up the stairs he laid down and refused to do any more. Giving me the look, like you crazy lady, you are just going to come back up here again. I will wait for you here. It is truly amazing how a twenty-pound dog can make himself weigh fifty pounds when he doesn't want to do something. So now I do my flights of stairs by myself with my dog shaking his head at me waiting for me to get down and do something really fun like chase him around the kitchen table trying to get his toy. Point being, find what fun is for you! Do *something* daily!

At the first Reverse Button Retreat we had yoga available for those who wanted to try it first thing in the morning. Now I have learned there are many types of yoga out there and many types of instructors, so I encourage you to shop around to find your right match if you decide to go down this route. Since the retreat was all people who had back pain, I chose a beginner Hatha yoga class that was for back pain. I chose two different instructors so the participants can see how it can be different with different people. I loved the response from one of the guys in the group who had never tried yoga before. He was shocked at how hard it was for his body and then equally shocked at how good he felt after. They were all blown away to find out that there were so many free resources on YouTube, and they couldn't use the excuse of not wanting to drive to the gym anymore. We talked about the importance of whatever exercise program that you try to make sure to listen to your body. I extended my arm as an example and said see, if you try to overstretch your body has a reflex called the "stretch reflex" that is there to keep you from hyperextension. It is there to protect you. If you push past this, you could hurt yourself. Pain is not always gain! I then asked if anyone remembered a toy I had as a child that we called a "Chinese finger torture," they all nodded. I said, remember you had to relax in to actually be able to get your fingers out." They all nodded again. I said so if you can work just to the point that you are not fighting the body or you cave in and create a slack in the body, generally you will actually achieve more range of motion and I extended my arm to show the difference. They were all amazed. If you'd like me to send you videos or additional reference material not able to be published with the book, just email at: ReverseButton-Book@gmail.com with the subject, "Additional Content."

CHAPTER

9

Why It's so Hard to Get Rid of Back Pain

S o, why is it so hard to get rid of back pain and avoid surgery? I feel that it comes down to realizing that we are a holistic being, not segmented like much of the world wants to describe us and any issues we are dealing with. Having a paradigm shift, you can find comfort within your discomfort. That by celebrating all is working well in your body you actually release chemicals that help support the body to heal. That by having a paradigm shift that you now recognize that the body wants to work from comfort and function, is huge! This mindset shift alone is monumental. To have the recognition that when you are in pain it is often the body's communication tool to say, "Hey, something is going on here, physically, mentally, emotionally, or spiritually" and that numbing it out or trying to "be tough" and ignore it is no longer serving us well. To recognize that the answer to how to avoid surgery and get rid of back pain so you can live a full "funspan" of life is all inside of you. It may need support, but the key elements are there!

A common term I say to my clients all the time (and I get giddy when I hear them say it themselves in a story) is, "Yeah, body!" Celebrating what is working well and when the body does hit the Reverse Button and finds its way back to its best comfort and function! One of my favorite stories I love to share is about recognition of the vagus nerve. When I was going through my training at the Rocky Mountain Ortho-Bionomy Center in Denver, about halfway through the two-year program I was in my prime of taking care of myself. I was eating really well, I was doing cardio about an hour a day, five times a week. My blood work looked amazing and yet I was gaining about a pound or two a week. So much that I had gained over fifty pounds. My doctor was stumped. She said that the only thing she had left to suggest was that I move up to seven days a week in my exercise. This seems ridiculous to me. If I wasn't maintaining with what I was doing, it had to be something else.

I went to my first trauma class and learned about the sympathetic and parasympathetic nervous systems. For simplification: the flight-or-fight system and the vagus nerve. In that weekend class I had about eight to ten hours of work either directly or indirectly supporting my body to find its Reverse Button back to a time that the vagus nerve was not stuck on. You know if your vagus is locked on if you resonate with this comment: "I feel like I am running around with my foot on the gas and break at the same time." If this is not you, you may know someone like this. I had been diagnosed with PTSD, adrenal fatigue, blowing out my adrenals, and cortisol flooding. The vagus nerve is our tenth brain nerve and it connects our brain with all our organs. It is designed to regulate their function so we can either fight or run away. It is originally there for us to flee from the Saber tooth Lion and then shut back off again – not stay on forever. At the beginning of the class we watched a deer in the woods get startled and then run off and shake, then go about its day grazing peacefully in a field. In our society today, most of us don't take the time to shake. We stack the stress inside, one issue after another until the body is fully frozen inside and it presents itself as a dis-ease or debilitating pain, especially in the back.

At the end of the first weekend of work on my vagus nerve, I had lost about ten pounds and my Reverse Button had been found. I started losing weight just as easily as it had come on about one to two pounds a week. Then my husband and I went on a trip to New Zealand to look for retirement property (he was a dual citizen). We were in the South Island on a narrow gravel road and in a camper van when a fully loaded log truck came screaming down the mountain side and he pulled to the edge. All I could see was the ocean very far down the cliff below. Wisely, my vagus went into full action. I was upset and scared and my husband was offended that I didn't trust in his driving abilities. He was confident of where the edge of the road was. We drove on and it happened a second time. I told him to pull over. I got out of the car and used a self-care technique to drain my adrenals and to bring me back into present time. I walked; I took deep breaths. I came back to the van and declared that I didn't want a retirement property on this road and that we should go explore another area. He said OK and turned the van around. About ten minutes into the drive, he turned to me and said, "You are better?" "Yep," I said. "We are going the other way." We had been together for about sixteen years at this point so he knew my patterns pretty well. "No, you are better in minutes, usually something like that would have you jacked up for days." I got so geeked-out excited. "My vagus nerve is working!" It was my first time of really being able to feel a difference.

I am pretty sure looking back at my life that I may have spent more time with my vagus turned on; but the truly amazing thing is that it did find its way back to calm, to function; even if it had to search back to conception for the Reverse Button! So, what does it look like when the body lets go of trauma? It can look like shaking like the deer, it can look like body jerks, electrical sensations throughout the body, unprovoked tears or laughter, and sudden changes in body temperature either hot or cold. When we are looping in trauma, we can't feel these things. Trauma likes to release out the extremities (arms and legs) primarily, and if they are blocked, they can get creative. I had a client who came to me for the first time after a knee surgery. She was really upset that she was developing restless leg syndrome. We saw each other a few times and then she screamed out mid-session, "There it is! It is happening now!" Before this she couldn't fully recognize when it would happen because it felt so random to her. Now it was clear. Her body was trying to be brilliant and release the trauma from the surgery but it was having to push everything through the other leg. I helped her body find a reflexive rhythm so it the gift of those times with my sister. She and I shared a bed until I was in the second grade and a room until I was in high school. My nervous system knows her as a safe place and vice versa. While we live miles apart; when we are together (and even over the phone at times) we create the opportunity for release and it's big! Yeah, body!

I'm happy to share more content with you about the vagus nerve and more that wasn't able to be put in the book, just email me at: ReverseButtonBook.com.

CHAPTER

10

Living Your Whole Life Fully to Its Best Comfort and Function

I am deeply grateful that you have come on this journey with me to find your whole self and to learn to honor the intelligence that is in your whole being! Recently there was a post on Facebook that was going around asking people to post their first picture and their most recent picture side by side. For most of us, we have been on Facebook for about nine or ten years now. When I stopped and really looked at where I was before this journey of exploration for my own health and for others I was blown away. Many people commented on how much better I look now. I posted my pictures saying, "I'm aging like a fine wine! It's just getting better all the time!" I truly believe this is true not only for me but those whom I work with on a regular basis. This is the Reverse Button.

In this book, I have tried to share many stories and bits of information I have collected in this journey to date. I do believe in being a full-time student of life and so I know there is more for us to discover going forward both together and individually. Sometimes I will be introduced to someone at an event and asked to help them because as they flew in, they got a stabbing pain in the back and are so uncomfortable. I work with them for only a few minutes and I hear back months later that just a few minutes of work profoundly changed a bigger issue going on in their life. It always blows me away and humbles me.

I loved it a few months ago when I was at a convention in Phoenix and a security guard was called because they believed that someone I was working with had too much to drink and was passed out. We all had a good laugh when we assured the security guard that honestly, she hadn't been drinking, she was just so relaxed as I worked on her upper back and shoulders.

I am grateful for my friend who called me the day after a session and said, "I don't know what you did but I had the craziest dream last night after you worked on my arm and told me that it was connected to an issue with my gut. In the dream my arm was sawed off and I was being beat with it and told that I shouldn't drink Diet Cola anymore. I got up and dumped all my pop down the drain and noticed my arm was in full function again." When she shared her story, I reminded her that I never told her what to eat or drink, I had just helped her make the connection of the gut and her arm pain and had worked with her third-eye to bring fresh blood flow so she could have clarity. I set the environment, and her amazing self put the pieces together to give her the information for her to live in her best comfort and function. Yeah, body!

I wish I had recorded a client who came to see me for swelling in her legs and in her second session she mentioned that since the swelling was better, she wanted to know what else we could work on. We decided to see if there was an option for her body to avoid a recommended knee surgery. When we she got off the table, her eyes got wide. She declared, "My knees feel better!" And then proceeded to throw her arms up in the air and do a victory lap around the table, as if she was in the movie *Rocky!* It was glorious what her body was able to do in one session! It found its Reverse Button back to its comfort and function! Yeah, body!

I am grateful when I have the opportunity to see people overtime, like what happened in this book, we get to truly grow and learn about your body as it is in this chapter of your life and invite a new one to start. One client that has been seeing me since the beginning of the Ortho Healing Center, embodies this so deeply. We started for her lack of function in her back and now she has awareness of herself, her system, her gifts, and her challenges. She knows when she needs outside support and she has a large tool bag of internal support she can lean into. She knows her Reverse Button!

We talked a lot at the Reverse Button Retreat that each person came to the event with an idea that they were there to fix their problem. They were focused on their one main problem. My guess, this was true of you too when you purchased this book. It is my dream for you now, that like the participants of the first retreat, you now know it is so much more than your one problem. That you are a whole, perfect human being that is a full system from the physical to the energetic and have new tools to support your body in finding its Reverse Button back to your best comfort and function in a whole way. It is my dream for you that, just like Mr. Texas shared in his exit interview, he felt like a Frankenstein before: separate, clunky parts and now they are whole and calm together. Yeah, body! Yeah, you!

As this book comes to a close, it is my hope that you share your new knowledge with others. You share this book with others. And if you decide that you want more, because there is always more; you will contact me at ReverseButtonBook@gmail.com and we will find your best way to get what you need. You are your own best advocate for your health. You know your body best. You know who needs to be in your tool bag for support for you to live your best life of comfort and function. If that is me, let's talk and I would be honored to facilitate and support you to hitting your Reverse Button together and living your whole life to its best comfort and function!

Acknowledgments

This book was made possible by such a collection of experiences and people to thank, it is difficult to even know where to start and ultimately, I am confident I will end up leaving someone out by accident. I often say my superpower is to collect and connect people. I am truly blessed to have collected the most amazing tribe in my life of supporters who believe, encourage, and inspire me daily. I thank each and every one of you!

Being a member of Team Global, who is a collaborative of business partners with a servant's heart, inspired me to read personal development daily and set my word for the year to be "both!" Many years ago, I learned the value of having choice, but it is only recently that I am aware of the concept of "both." It was this concept that opened me to watch the webinar that led me to write this book with The Author Incubator Program. I had dreamed of writing since I was eleven years old when I won my first writing contest. A cabin has sat on my vision board for years to represent the year that I will take off from my life to go and write my first book. Thanks to The Author Incubator and the concept of "both," I realized I didn't need to wait to write. I could do it alongside my life now and reach more people to help with my unique work at the same time. Then as this book unfolded a new option of retreats emerged; a business partner in Team Global reached out and asked if I could come to Idaho to do a retreat and share the book. I jumped online to find a location and the first one that came up was nearly identical to the cabin that was on my vision board. Of course, this book was to be written now and the cabin came, in a better way than my limited imagination had originally put together.

I am a believer of mentorship and feel this is an important place to thank my three biggest mentors of my life: Sheri Covey of the Rocky Mountain Ortho-Bionomy Center, John Ryan of Team Global, and Mia Hewett author of *Meant For More*. Each of you has encouraged me to grow in many ways, and modeled a life for me to stretch, to think, to trust, and be my full self! Thank you all from the bottom of my heart!

I want to say a deep-hearted thank you to all of my clients of the Ortho Healing Center and particularly those who experienced the first Reverse Button Retreat and those who attended the first 8-week online program with me. Your trust in our work together is what makes this book accessible for so many to see themselves in the stories and hopefully have that moment: if it helped her, maybe it can help me too! You are truly the heroes of this book!

My acknowledgments couldn't be complete without mentioning the two beings that share my house and my heart on a daily basis: my daughter Victoria, and my dog and business partner: L.D. These two have been impacted most by the writing of this book. As I write this, L.D. patiently sits at the end of the couch with his favorite teddy bear waiting for any moment I will look up from the computer and take a break to play with him. He is a constant being of light and love for both me and the clients of the Ortho Healing Center. Victoria has cheered me on daily to follow through with this dream. She has given me space and quiet in the house to write when I needed it, and was my right-hand gal through my first retreat making sure all guests were extremely well taken care of that added an important element to the whole experience.

Thank You

T hank you for going on this journey with me to supporting you in finding your Reverse Button back to fully living your life again! As a thank you to my readers I have created bonus content of quick one-page reference sheets and videos of many of the self-care techniques that I have talked about in the book. Email: ReverseButtonBook@gmail.com with the subject line: "BONUS CONTENT" and I will send you this bonus material valued at over $500 for FREE as my thank you!

About the Author

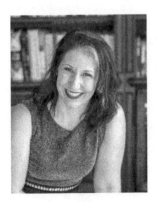

Practitioner Abby Beauchamp is the Owner of the Ortho Healing Center, opened in 2012 in Portland, Oregon. She blends her passion and background in Montessori experiential education and natural healthcare together to provide a unique environment for healing the whole being from the physical to the energetic. Her clinic empowers humans, dogs, and horses, to find their best comfort and function.

As a former Montessori school founder and administrator, Abby learned the value of scientific observation, and to honor and be in awe of the intelligence of human development and how environment can play a major role in that development beyond the limitations of the teacher.

In 2010, she worked with horses through experiential groundwork workshops offered at Natural Whisperings™ in Canby, Oregon where she learned to appreciate the intelligence of these great beings and recognize the communication through the energetic field.

In 2012, Abby attended her first Ortho-Bionomy class taught by Zarna Carter of Australia; where she got the vision to someday travel and teach throughout the world! This first class was for both humans and horses. Shortly after the first class, she enrolled with Sheri Covey, in the Practitioner Training Program through the Rocky Mountain Ortho-Bionomy® Center, and received her practitioner designation two years later. She continues to work with them today to deepen her understanding and grow as a practitioner and to date has completed over 1500 hours of training in Ortho-Bionomy.

In 2013, Abby became a pioneer for Ortho-Bionomy in Oregon. She worked with the state to change the laws recognizing Ortho-Bionomy as a safe, unique bodywork practice under the oversight of the Society of Ortho-Bionomy International®.

In recent years, Abby has expanded the Wellness Center to also include business mentorship, Intuitive Healing Facilitation, Reverse Button™ Programs, remote and online services. As a forever student of life, Abby, and the Ortho Healing Center continue to grow and expand services and connections to empower all in living their best comfort and function! To receive additional content valued at over $500 that we could not put in this book, email us at: ReverseButtonBook@gmail.com with the subject line, "Additional Content".